The Drug Awareness Library™

Danger:
COCAINE

Ruth Chier

The Rosen Publishing Group's
PowerKids Press™
New York

Published in 1996 by The Rosen Publishing Group, Inc.
29 East 21st Street, New York, NY 10010

First Edition

Book design: Erin McKenna

Photo credits: Cover by Michael Brandt; pp. 4, 16, 19 by Maria Moreno; p. 7 © Bertrand Rieger/Gamma Liaison; pp. 8, 11, 12 Sarah Friedman; p. 15 © Chad Ehlers/International Stock; p. 20 by Lauren Piperno.

Chier, Ruth.
    Danger: cocaine / Ruth Chier
        p.   cm. — (The drug awareness library)
    Includes index.
    Summary: Describes how cocaine is made and the dangers of using it.
    ISBN 0-8239-2337-1
    1. Cocaine habit—Juvenile literature. 2. Cocaine—Juvenile literature. [1. Cocaine habit. 2. Cocaine.]
I. Title. II. Series.
HV5810.C54 1996
362.29'8—dc20   96-7862
                                                                                        CIP
                                                                                         AC

Manufactured in the United States of America

Contents

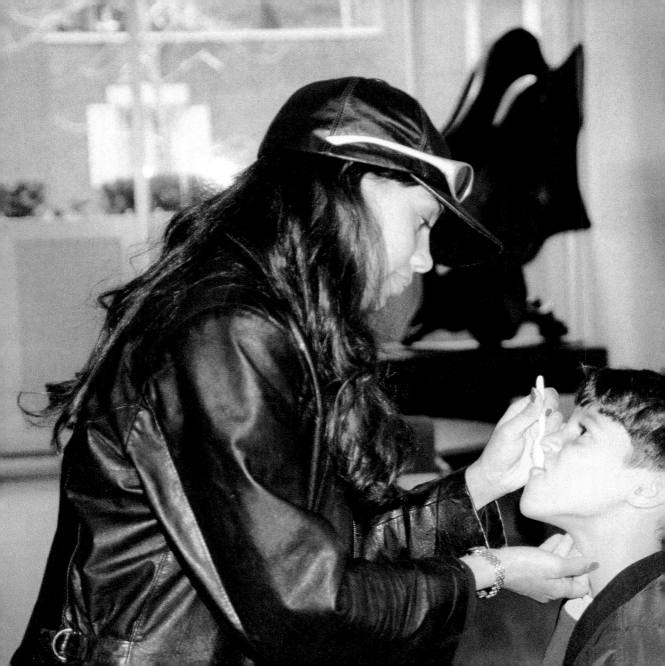

What Is a Drug?

A drug is a **chemical** (KEM-ih-kul) that changes the way you think and feel and act. Some drugs help your body. These drugs are called medicines. They are usually given to you by your parent or a doctor. Medicine will help you get well if you are sick.

Other drugs are dangerous and can hurt your body. They are usually **illegal** (il-LEE-gul). Some people use illegal drugs anyway. **Cocaine** (ko-KAYN) is an illegal drug.

◀ Some drugs, like medicine, help your body get well.

5

What Is Cocaine?

Cocaine comes from the coca plant. Coca plants grow in South America. The leaves of the plant are picked. Then they are crushed and mixed with two chemicals. Some people call cocaine "coke" or "snow" because it is a white powder.

Cocaine speeds up a person's body. It is a kind of **stimulant** (STIM-yoo-lent). Stimulants make a person's heart and brain work faster.

Coca plants grow in the Andes ▶
Mountains of South America.

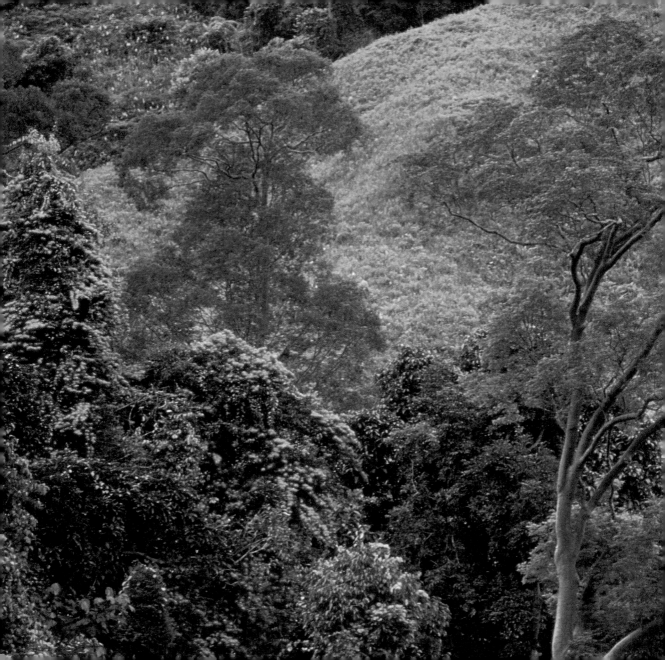

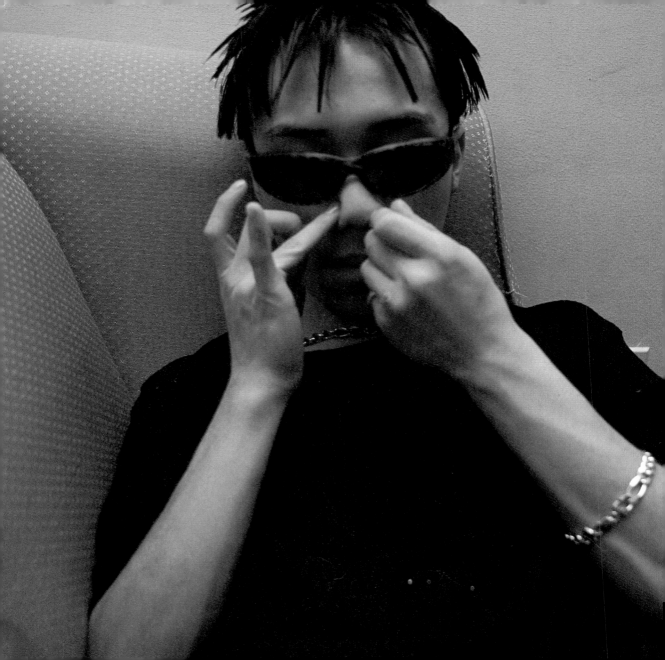

How Is Cocaine Used?

Cocaine is usually snorted through a person's nose. The fine powder gets into a person's **bloodstream** (BLUD-streem) quickly through the tiny veins in a person's nose. Some people **inject** (in-JEKT) cocaine. Others smoke it in a form called crack.

No matter how it is used, cocaine is dangerous. Some people die the first time they try it.

◄ Snorting cocaine hurts the inside of a person's nose.

9

Getting High

When a person uses cocaine, she gets "**high**" (HY). She has lots of energy and feels wide awake. She may also feel jumpy and restless. She feels strong and smart. She feels like she can do anything. But those feelings only last for a little while. Then they go away. That person is left feeling **depressed** (dee-PREST), sleepy, and sick to her stomach. She wants to make the bad feelings go away by getting high again.

When a person's high goes away, ▶
he or she feels sad and sick.

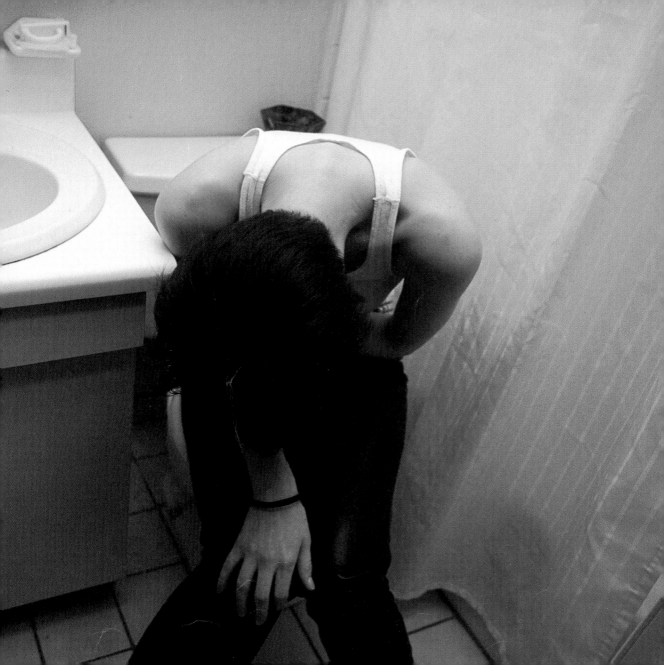

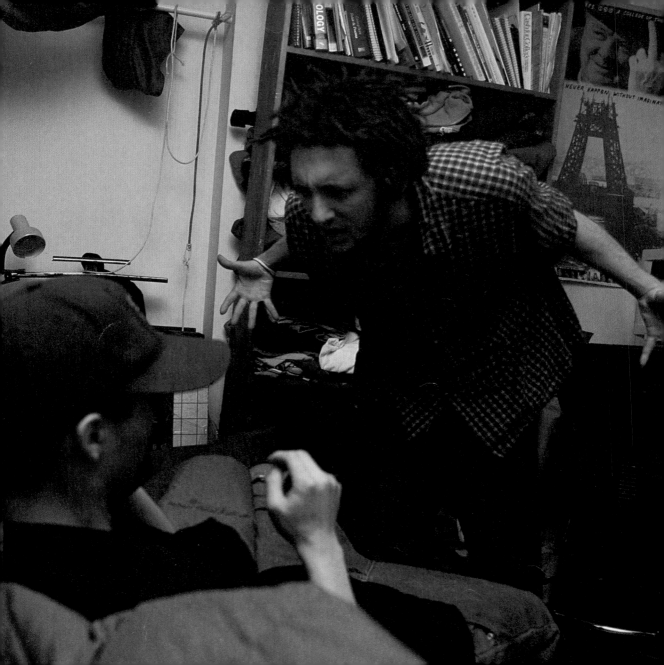

Drugs Change a Person

When a person uses cocaine, his life changes. He stops caring about his friends and family. He doesn't go to school or to soccer practice. He may stop eating and sleeping. He may be cranky or jumpy. He may get angry a lot, and may even get violent. He may have a hard time focusing on anything but getting his next high.

◄ It can be scary when someone who is on cocaine gets angry or violent.

Why Do People Use Cocaine

Some people use cocaine because they think it is fun or exciting. Others use it because it makes them feel grown-up. Some people try it because their friends do.

Some people use cocaine to run away from problems in their lives. When they are high, they may forget about their problems. But using cocaine makes a person have more problems.

Kids often try new activities because their friends do them. It is the same way with drugs. ▶

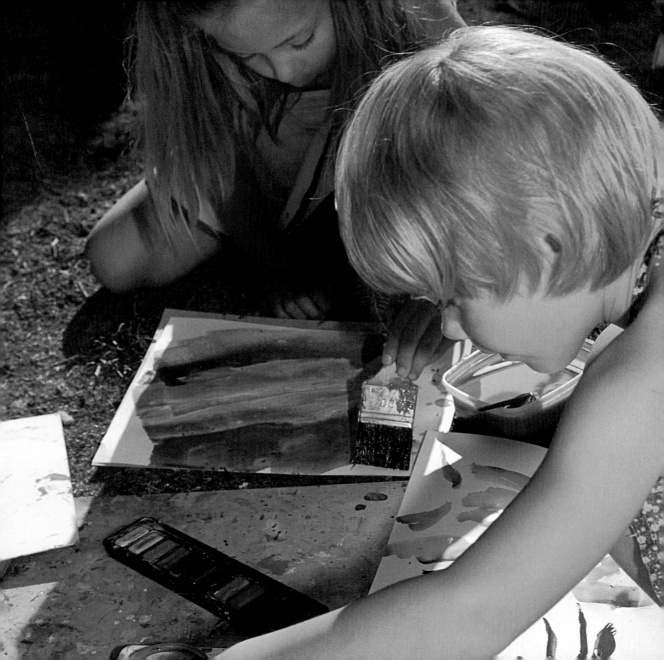

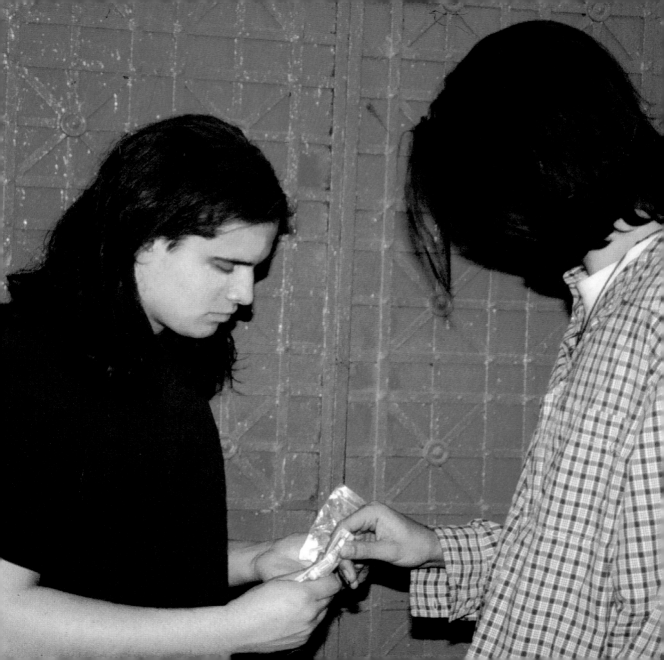

Addiction

Many people who use cocaine become **addicted** (a-DIK-ted) to it. Some people are addicted after trying cocaine for the first time. Having an addiction means being **dependent** (dee-PEN-dent) on a drug. Cocaine addicts like feeling high. But they feel depressed when the drug wears off. They believe they can get rid of that feeling by using cocaine to get high again.

Once a person is addicted to cocaine, he will do anything he can to get high.

◀ A person who is addicted to cocaine will do whatever he has to do to get more of the drug.

Cocaine Addicts

People who are addicted to drugs are called **addicts** (AD-dikts). Cocaine addicts think that they need cocaine more than they need food, water, and sleep. Today, over 115,000 teens in the United States are addicted to cocaine.

There are many places a cocaine addict can go for help. She can talk to a parent, a teacher, or a minister. She can also call a drug hotline, and someone will talk to her about getting help.

Cocaine addicts would rather have the drug than food. ▶

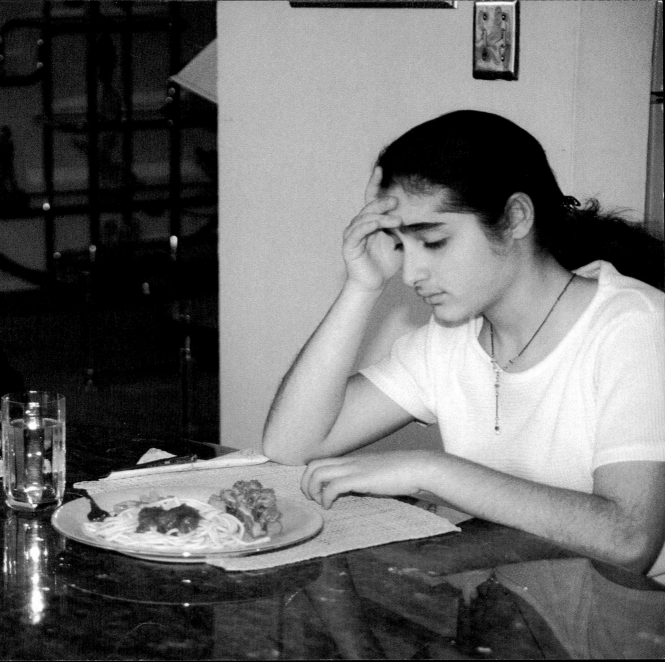

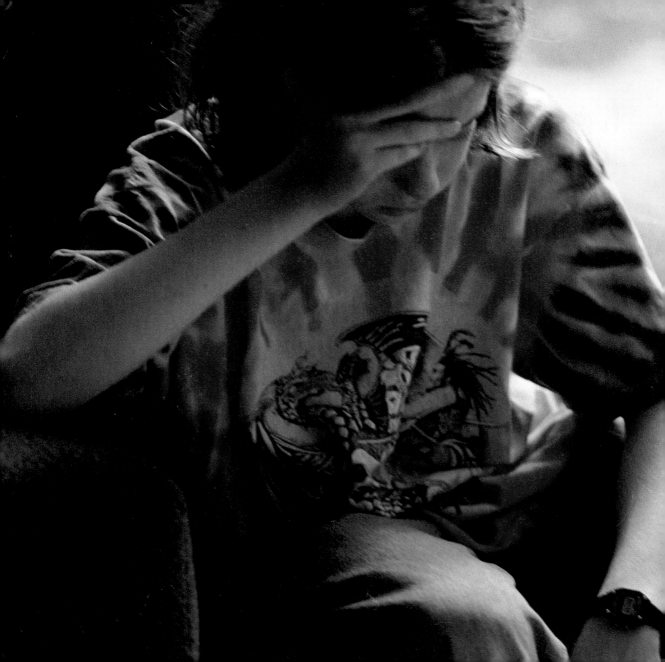

Cocaine and Crime

Many crimes are committed by people who are on drugs, or who need money to buy more drugs. Cocaine is an expensive drug. Cocaine addicts begin to need the drug more often. They often run out of money to buy it. So they steal money. A cocaine addict may steal from his family or friends. Or he may rob stores. Then the addict has two problems: his addiction and his crimes. Cocaine affects the user and everyone around him.

◀ Using cocaine doesn't solve problems in a person's life. It only makes new ones.

Taking Care of Yourself

If someone, even a friend, asks you to try cocaine, you can say no. It is up to you to decide what you put in your body. Be smart and take care of yourself. Using cocaine is not fun. It can ruin your life. If someone offers you cocaine at school or in your neighborhood, tell your teacher, principal, or parent.

Cocaine hurts the lives of people who use it. You don't want it to hurt yours.

Glossary

addict (AD-dikt) Person who can't control his or her use of a drug.

addicted (a-DIK-ted) Unable to control the use of a drug.

bloodstream (BLUD-streem) Blood flowing through the body.

chemical (KEM-ih-kul) Building block from which things are made.

cocaine (ko-KAYN) Drug made from the coca plant that is changed into white powder.

dependent (dee-PEN-dent) Relying on a drug to feel normal.

depressed (dee-PREST) Feeling very sad.

high (HY) Feeling of false happiness that a person gets when he uses a drug.

illegal (il-LEE-gul) Against the law.

inject (in-JEKT) Using a needle to put a drug into your body.

stimulant (STIM-yoo-lent) Drug that speeds up your body.

Index